DATING FOR WOMEN

A Social Bible for Women to find
Themselves and their Soulmates

Table of Contents

INTRODUCTION

"Men, you can't live with them, you can't live without them."

This is one of the most common phrases uttered by women when it comes to men and their relationships. Another phrase as well as a book title is "Men are from Mars, Women are from Venus."

When we look at these title and statements, a picture begins to form in our minds and preconceived notions begin to cloud our vision and build up our expectations when it comes to relationships. For men, their initial thinking in general is, "Wow, she's hot. I need to go and get me some of that" or "She's sexy. I want to go home with her tonight."

When we investigate the male mindset, we will see that most of the time they are thinking about sex or some activity or situation that could possibly lead to sex. For women, however, their thinking is different. When we explore the mind of a woman, she is typically looking at a male as a possible provider for her and their children as well as protection from the dangers of the world.

With this being said, we aren't ruling out that women are sexual beings as well. In fact, when a woman finds the right man or someone that she is compatible with, engaging in a sexual and physical intimate relationship is just as satisfying if not more so.

However, the biggest question that we need to address is how does a woman find that perfect man and what does she need to do to keep him?

This is why I wrote this book. I wanted to write it as a practical guide for woman to understanding themselves and others. In this guide, we will focus on questions that every woman may have when it comes to dating. We will also dive into areas of self-worth and offer advice for woman to use in the modern age.

As we approach the year 2020, it is more important than ever for women to take control of their lives and understand their internal values. When dating, they need to know that they oversee the situation and that there is someone out there for everyone.

When you complete this book, I want you to take away something. I want you to take away information that you can apply to your life and your personal situation. I believe that with a little help and a little guidance, we all can be happy.

CHAPTER ONE
Building on you – Preparing for the Dating World

When it comes to dating, many people start at an early age. At around thirteen, fourteen years old, men and women begin to physically change. They enter a period of life known as puberty. It is when they enter this stage, they begin to take an interest in the opposite sex. This interest will lead to dating and then beyond.

One of the hardest parts of this time of life is that our minds and our physical bodies tell us what to do separately. For the next several years, our brains and our bodies won't work well together and the choices we make as well as the perceptions that we have will be skewed. This is why before you jump into dating or if you have been dating for a while now, you may want to take a step back and focus on you and not a lifelong relationship.

Treat Yourself Like the "PRIZE" You Really Are

When considering dating or entering any type of relationship be it with a man, woman, friend or whatever, you need to treat yourself like a prize. Now, when it comes to treating yourself as a prize, I am not talking about acting like you are the greatest thing since sliced bread or that you are better than anyone or everyone else. In fact, I mean the exact opposite.

I am referring to treating yourself with respect and not allowing anyone else to determine your self-worth or innate value. When entering into relationships with others, women have a tendency to focus more with their hearts and their emotions. When we focus on our hearts and emotions, we tend to take rash actions or see things that are not there.

One example would be when you find yourself in an abusive relationship. Women who find themselves in an abusive relationship may believe that they deserve what they are getting because they are the problem. Women will look at the man they are with as the most important thing in the world because they started off so sweet and loving and over time, began to change and assert their dominance over them. In these situations, women will typically begin to believe that their self-worth is not valid and stop thinking of themselves as a prize but rather a consolation prize or the gift that gets re-gifted no one wants.

Therefore, you need to have a healthy mental attitude and a foundation of your own self-worth. If you don't have this self-worth, then no man will see your value and assign you the value they perceive you are worth.

Self-Respect and Personal Boundaries

The foundation for treating yourself as the prize is having self-respect for yourself and determining your personal boundaries. The first thing that we will talk about is self-respect.

Self-Respect

Point blank, if you don't have self-respect and care about your personal self, no one else will either. When it comes to creating self-respect, it starts with creating a mental avatar of yourself. When we create a mental avatar, we have a point of reference to relate to. Too often women will create mental avatars based on pictures they see on TV, in movies, in ads that constantly tell them what is acceptable in society and if you don't fit into this societal mold, you will not be loved, and you are not worth anything to anyone else.

Therefore, women need to find strong personal role models and realistic avatars to model after. In the past several years, you have begun to see women are getting more realistic role models. You see them in television, movies, in politics and even in the classrooms. This influx of female role models is a great thing and is a positive start for finding and understanding what self-respect really means.

Personal Boundaries

The topic of personal boundaries and acting against those who violate those boundaries has been running hot in the media over the past several months. As I write this book, the "Me Too" movement is growing strong and women who have been suffering in silence for decades are now finally speaking out over the violations of their personal boundaries and making those who have violated them take responsibility for their actions.

When it comes to creating personal boundaries, it is vital that you hold strong to these boundaries and enforce your decision at every turn. If you encounter pressure from others either on a personal level or from those in authority, it is vital that you hold strong to your personal boundaries and call out those who violate them.

Tap into your Authentic Self

We are all strong individuals. We are all unique and we all have something of value to offer not only to ourselves but to others as well. This is important that we know, understand, and can tap into our authentic selves. So, what exactly is our authentic self?

Our authentic self is the person we let out when we are alone. This is the person we see in the mirror when we wake up and the person we act like when we are alone. Too often we try to put on a mask or face of someone we are not just to impress someone else. The problem with this is that we are not allowing people to know who we really are. If we hide our authentic selves too long and are afraid to be ourselves then we are doing just as much damage to a relationship and to ourselves then giving into fear.

Don't Compromise or Settle

The final piece of advice I wanted to give you in this chapter is probably the most important. When dating or finding a relationship, you don't want to compromise or settle. When you are out there, be out there. Find several people to talk to and interact with. The odds are that the first person that you come across won't be Mr. Right.

When we begin dating, our mental mindset tells us that we need to find the perfect mate on the first attempt. 99% of the time this will never happen. When we meet someone, and it is going well, we will believe that this person is perfect or that we can never do any better. We will then focus on our biological clock and with every passing month believe that we are getting farther and farther way from starting a family.

Therefore, we don't want to compromise and settle for what we have or what we feel is our best option. When we do settle or compromise, we will eventually find ourselves in a situation where we find that perfect person and are trapped in a situation that will hurt more people than it will help. Often those who settle will quickly become bored and go in search of others to scratch the itch.

So, take your time, see what is out there, build your relationships and when it is right, it is right.

CHAPTER TWO
How the Past Will Affect Your Future

"You are what you eat."
"Monkey See, Monkey Do"

These two sayings are a good reflection on our mental health and development when we are growing up. When we are children, our minds are clear slates, a blank canvas for us to build the person we want to be. We are very curious and want to learn and explore the world around us.

When we are babies, we rely on our parents to accomplish this task. When we see our parents hugging and kissing, we imprint in our minds that this is an acceptable behavior and as such, we will learn this behavior and reproduce it to become accepted by and fit in with the world around us. The same goes for bad behaviors as well. I remember when my daughter was two or three years old, and she was sitting in the back of the car making the gestures of her smoking. Now, of course she didn't know what she was doing, and the behavior was innocent, but on the other hand, it was a learned behavior that she saw from the actions of her parents.

Adult Dating Life

When we embark on our adult dating life, the interactions between our parents in front of as well as behind closed doors affects us and our future relationships. For example, if we are laying in our beds in the middle of the night and we begin to hear our parents argue and fight then this becomes engrained in our subconscious of acceptable activity.

If we see that this shouting escalates into physical violence such as slapping, pushing or worse than we begin to accept it as true and will draw upon it later in life. On the other side of the coin, if we see that our parents are in loving relationships, there is no shouting or violence then it is generally engrained that this is acceptable behavior and we will not act out or seek out violent or inappropriate relationships.

The Father Figure

When it comes to relationships, women will typically, but not always, drift towards men who fill a father figure role. Now, if the woman's father was violent or abusive then they will drift towards a violent or abusive partner. If their father was loving and caring, then they will drift more towards that type of partner.

There is a third option as well. Depending on the woman's personal self-worth or avatar they may move towards the opposite of their father. For example, they may break the cycle of violence and find someone that will not harm them like their parent did. Also, if their father figure was absent from their lives, they drift towards a distant type male partner that may not be physically or emotionally violent or abusive but rather is someone they will settle for since they don't have a real male role model to model.

Building a strong Childhood

Therefore, building and nurturing a strong childhood for women as well as men is vital to the future health and well-being of their relationships. If a woman has a strong male role model growing up, she will know what to expect as well as know what is accepted in a loving relationship. When it comes to a man, you will also get what you put into it. A man that knows how to treat a woman like a prize and not a trophy to be displayed is what you should look for because you deserve to be respected.

If you as a woman or a man find that you are in or were in a childhood relationship with your parents that tainted your future relationships, you need to seek out counseling and work through issues that are preventing you from finding that loving stable relationship. Put you first and then US second.

CHAPTER THREE
How You Choose To Date

In the first two chapters of this book, I wanted to give you the foundation that you need to create a positive mindset for your love and dating life. If you continue through this book without first reading and understanding the mental aspects and fixing any issues that you find in your life then you will not have as successful a love life and dating success that you could have had if you had just taken the time to really understand yourself before understanding someone else.

I and I Alone will Determine my Dating Preferences and How I will be Treated

When it comes to dating, you need to know your self-worth. After you have determined and created a positive self-worth image, you need to start building the image of your perfect mate. This is where you and you alone will determine your dating preferences and who stacks up to them.

When choosing your dating style, many outsiders will have their own opinions on your relationships. For example, your parents or co-workers will say, "Girl, you know I have the perfect guy for you. He is tall, dark, handsome, has money, and will treat you right."

When you have people in your life that like to set people up, you want to be cautious. What people look like on the outside or the avatar that they project typically isn't what they are in real life.

When people try to be flashy or show the world how good they are, they are typically trying to create an internal self-worth based on others' opinions. This type of relationship will typically never work out, so stay clear. However, you might get a nice meal out of it, so roll the dice.

Others' Opinions and the Double Standard

This is a big one when it comes to determining your dating preferences. Typically, women live in a man's mind when thinking about dating and relationships. There's an old saying:

"A Cook in the Kitchen"

"A Maid in the house"

"A Whore in the Bedroom"

When dating, the one thing that you can expect is for others to put their nose in where it doesn't belong. I like to say, "If you are going to give me your two cents, write a check." As I look back at my dating life, I am amazed as to how many people would tell me how things should work and why things didn't work out for them. When I look back at these situations, I was amazed at how many people preached on topics and situations they themselves never lived. And worse of all, talked themselves up to make you believe they were all that and a bag of chips.

Looking at this specific situation in dating, many men believe that you should be all focused on them. If you are not focused on them and have an opinion, then you are a slut. When it comes to women looking at you and your relationships, they may call you a whore or something along those lines because you don't fit into their vision or mold of a good person.

This is where your self-worth, avatar and desires will play a critical part. If you give in to these comments, and avatar images others create, you will never be happy. You need to really focus on you and your desire. It is vital that you distance yourself from negative people and really build a support group and community of likeminded people. When you can do this, you will have the pull of positive people and that Mr. Right should be in the bunch.

CHAPTER FOUR
Ready to find Mr. Right

Now that we have worked on ourselves and have determined what it is we want out of a relationship, it is now time to jump in with both two feet and see what we come up with when looking for Mr. Right.

Dating Advice for Women of All Ages

#1 – Just Chill

When it comes to dating, you don't need to focus on the perfect guy. What you want to do is find a "like." It can be their hair, eyes, smile, or overall attitude. When you find this like, go ahead and make the first move. If they are interested, suggest hanging out and having a little fun. After the first date or gathering, however you want to classify it, you can repeat the process, go in search for someone else or both. Just chill out and enjoy the moment. If you go too deep into the dating process "Getting Married at First Sight" as it were, you are robbing yourself of the entire process. So Just Chill!

#2 – Don't Change your Appearance

This is very important. When dating, you don't want to start off with the wrong impression or lead others to believe you are who you really aren't. Too often than not, people will do something crazy or out of character to impress a girl or a boy. One of the most common changes people will make is changing their appearance.

Now, when changing your appearance, I am not saying try to look nice or don't show off your key features. I am saying that you don't want to dress like a punk rock head banger if you are really a country girl at heart. The same goes for the other side of the coin. If you are a hard rocking heavy metal rocker, don't show up in a school girl outfit, unless that is the impression you want to give. You also do not need to dress up in a revealing outfit or show a lot of skin to impress a guy. Be yourself. If you feel comfortable in a pair of jeans and sneakers, wear them. It is important for your date to see the real you. Not a made-up image or an unrealistic perception of the perfect woman.

One great example of this is from the hit television program "Big Bang Theory." In one of the episodes, Raj and Howard go to a goth nightclub to pick up girls. They wear these tattoo sleeves, which I personally think are cool, to impress girls and make them think they are goth guys. At the end of the episode, they find themselves in a tattoo parlor going to get tattoos. When they were revealed, they didn't get what they were looking for.

The same goes for you and your appearance. If you find yourself going out of your way on a regular basis to change who you are inside as a person then you are not with the right person. If you want to change who you are because that is the person you want to be then all the power to you.

#3 – Don't Play the Chasing Game

This is something that can change your reputation and the overall tone of your relationships, so make sure that you choose wisely. There is a huge debate on if a woman should chase after a man or if a woman should just let a man chase after them. The truth is there isn't a clear-cut answer since each situation is different, but here is my opinion.

At the start of the relationship, don't chase after the man. This is my reasoning why. You want to hold on to your self-worth and your relationship avatar. When you have a man chase after you, you are opening their eyes to your self-worth. If they see that spark in your eyes and flutter in their hearts, then they will put in the effort to court you and see where the relationship will go. If you go after the man, typically, it is considered being desperate. This can be a negative in your relationships.

However, here is where the double standard rule comes in. If you are an older woman and you chase after a guy, it is considered sexy. I don't know why, but I guess when a man sees that you have experience as it were, it is more attractive and doesn't look as desperate if a younger woman did it. Sorry, not my rules.

#4 - Focus on What you CAN Control Not What you CAN'T Control

This is another huge factor when it comes to dating. When a woman enters a relationship, she will typically find one aspect of a man that she finds totally sexy and irresistible and overlook everything else.

Then after a month or so of dating, their true colors or aspects of his personality will shine through. This realization will quickly send the woman into "fix me" mode believing that their love is so strong that she can change him if she only had the chance.

If you find yourself in this type of relationship, run, run fast, and run far. When facing this situation, you need to focus on what you can change and control and not the aspects you can't.

When getting into a relationship, there will be a learning curve that you will both have to deal with. Throughout the years, we must deal with different areas of our lives. For example, our parents. As I stated previously in the book, how your parents act and how others in your immediate circle act will have a strong influence on how you see the world and live in it.

When we try to control situations that we just can't, we are doing ourselves a disservice. Trying to change others to fit your mold will only add stress and pressure to the relationship which will result in cheating, divorce, violence, or just overall resentment. If these happen and you have children or just find yourself in a situation you just can't get out of then what would you do next?

What you want to do is focus on you. You are the number one factor in this equation. You will want to make sure that you are educated, have a good job, a good home, money in the bank, and a positive outlook and attitude. If you don't have these things and you are in search of someone to change to fit your vision, you are destined to fail. Two messes don't make a match. Focus on yourself, be your perfect avatar, and everything else will fall into place.

#5 – Get Straight to the Point

Let's face it. We aren't getting any younger and if we are going to put in the time and energy into these guys, we need to get straight to the point and let them know where we stand. Now, I am not saying to drop your entire life story and tell them they need to the baby daddy. What I am saying is you need to get to the point and not play the cute school girl twirling her hair, chewing gum, and laughing at everything the guy says.

When getting to the point, you want to basically do that. You want to tell them that you are looking for a long-term relationship with a man who will want to have children. Of course, if this isn't what you want then by all means don't tell them that, but I believe you know what I mean.

Often women and men alike will just tell people what they want to hear or hide within themselves their true feelings. You see, it is always easier to hurt your own feelings and bottle up your own emotions than it is to hurt someone else.

However, when it comes to your life and your ultimate relationships, you are in total control. If you don't like the guy you're dating, then tell him that you're not interested in pursuing a long-term relationship. If you are in to him then make it known. It is important to know where each of you stands. Again, you want to be careful when you do this, however, it can totally blow up in your face on many levels. So, stay guarded, let yourself shine through and don't take the crap you don't deserve.

#6 – Personal Boundaries

We have talked about personal boundaries previously, but I wanted to go a little more into detail about this subject. When letting people know who you are and what you want, you also need to know where your personal boundaries are and make it known to all who may want to date you.

With personal boundaries, they can change from moment to moment, date to date. For example, where do you stand on kissing? When starting out in a relationship, the first serious form of physical contact is a kiss. When talking to your partner, you need to tell them where and when it is appropriate to kiss you and for how long.

Now, I don't want to start sounding like a broken record, but these are important subjects to discuss. If you don't want to be kissed, say no. If you want to be kissed, then let it be known. When creating your personal boundaries, don't be afraid of how others see you. If they don't respect these boundaries, they don't respect you. End of story.

#7 – Don't Dwell on Perfection

Another major thing you will have to learn is there is no such thing as perfection. I am not perfect, you are not perfect, and no one that you meet is perfect either. Another thing that you want to know is that imperfections are what make things perfect in the eyes of people who want to be with you. So, refer to tip #1. Chill out.

Final Tips

These are only a few tips that you can apply to your dating practices when looking for Mr. Right. Throughout the rest of the book, we will be adding more tips and advice that you can use. In the next chapter, we are going to focus on talking about men, what they want, and how you can use this information to spot the prince or the frog.

CHAPTER FIVE
Understanding Men 101

In this chapter, we are going to switch gears a little bit and instead of focusing on women, we are going to put men in the hot seat. When dating and building relationships, we must take the opposite sex into consideration not only for the health and well-being of a relationship but understanding men will allow women to know when they have found the right man and what to expect from them on many different levels.

What Men Want and How to be Treated

Just like women, men have specific needs and ways they want to be treated. Depending on the point of contact as well as stage of the personal relationship, different men will want and expect different things from women.

First, men want to be appreciated and feel that they are needed in a relationship. Since the beginning of time, man has had an evolutionary need to be the hunter, protector, and provider for the family. Since the first days of man, they have been going out hunting food, gathering what is needed for their family, and doing whatever they can to protect them.

In modern times, this ingrained primal instinct is still a part of our DNA. When a man meets a woman, their instinct is to be possessive and protective. Therefore, when men meet woman and they see them talking to other men, even though it is innocent, men will think dark and negative things. This results in difficulty for women to "play the field" with men when starting out in a relationship. Many men will instantly think that, "This is my woman, hands off" no matter if they just met, been going out for a short time, or are in a long-term relationship. Women need to be clear and upfront with men about their intentions. Don't drag men along, it will not end well.

Men and Sex

Okay, you knew we were going to talk about it, so let's just get it over with. Men want sex. Men love sex and if men aren't getting sex, they will go and find sex. In general, men and women think about sex in totally different ways. Again, this varies from individual to individual, but this is how sex is thought of between the genders.

Men – Men want the physical release when it comes to sex. They want the oral sex, they want the physical rush of having a woman perform sex on them, and they want the mental release of knowing they have sexually satisfied a woman. When the physical act of sex is over, men want to move on, in general like I said. They don't want to lay there and talk about their feelings or bond emotionally. Again, this is in general terms. There are a lot of men that do like this part of sex but not all.

Women and Sex

When it comes to sex for women, the general rule is the emotional connection over the physical connection. Now, this is not to say that women don't like the physical connection. In fact, many women will want the physical connection just as much if not more than men do. The main difference is that to become totally satisfied, women need the strength, security, and emotional support that sharing the physical with a man brings. In the emotional mind of a woman, sharing their body with a man is like sharing their soul. Therefore, women will seek out sex with others if they are not getting it from their partner. When asked, this is the number one reason why women cheat, "He wasn't there for me when I needed it."

Becoming More Patient and Understanding Towards Men

When you are going to get into a relationship with men, you really need to focus on becoming more patient and understanding with them. For those who aren't patient with men will quickly realize that they are jerks and will become unhappy with their relationships. Now, this is not to say that you shouldn't stand your ground or demand what you want out of a relationship, but you don't need to be an emotional mess either.

When being patient and understanding with men, you first need to realize that men are out for one thing. When a man typically meets a woman for the first time, they are doing so because they find a physical attraction towards them. For me, personal is in the eyes and the smile. For others, they are attracted to breasts, butts, the way they walk, their voice and even the little gestures they make. When men notice women, there is typically one thing that catches their attention and gets their blood pumping.

Once a man connects with a woman, the next thing that is going to be on their mind is sex. Yes, sex, I know it is a shocker, but sorry ladies, it is true. When men find a woman, the first thought that is going to go through their mind is what they are going to do during sex and how good it is going to be. By the time a man gets done with the first conversation with a woman, they have already imagined their first sexual encounter with you and are planning the next.

On the other side of the coin, when a woman typically meets a man, she will do the same thing. She will look at the man and find something that appeals to her. Again, it can be the eyes, smile, muscles, or butt. From there, she is looking at a man as a provider and how he would be towards her children if she currently had any or how he would be as a father to their children. Then she will start to think about how he would be in the sack.

When it comes to sex and the sexes, both men and woman when they meet will eventually turn to the point of sex. If a woman doesn't find a man sexy or can see herself having sex with a man, the man will enter what is known as the "Friends Zone." For a man who finds a woman physically attractive, this is the worst place to be.

Men Say Stupid Stuff

The next thing you need to know about men is that they tend to say a lot of stupid things. Sorry ladies, this is engrained in their DNA and can't be avoided. When a man says something stupid, it is because their male parts are talking to them over their brain.

When a man comes over to you in a bar or other locations and makes a move on you, it isn't because they are dumb, it is because they are trying to be cute and grab your attention.

When a man comes up to you and says, "Hey good looking, what's up? Can I buy you a drink?" It isn't their brain talking, it is their little friend or big friend in some cases. Therefore, many people, when getting a line like this think," Here's another loser."

This is where women must kick in their understanding gene. Women need to understand that men have no clue what they are saying in this moment and to excuse them. If at this point the woman sees that "spark," they should over look what they say and initiate the conversation. If they don't see the "spark," tell them something like, "Gas prices, but I saved enough money to buy myself a drink. Thanks for the offer, though."

Men are Possessive

This is not our fault. Well, some men are jerks and it is their fault, but in general it isn't. Like I said earlier, it is engrained in their DNA and just something you must deal with. When you find a possessive man, you need to set them straight right away. You want to let them know where you are emotionally in the relationship and what you are looking for. Tell them that you aren't looking for a man, but just looking to have fun. If they are not into it then you need to brush them aside now.

If you are a possessive man, it can be a good thing. It shows a woman that you are committed to a relationship. If, however, you are too possessive and won't allow them to make their own choices or you snap at the male waiter for asking her what she wants to order, then you have an issue that needs to be addressed right then and there.

Communication is KEY!

Ladies, men are not mind readers. One of the most annoying things for a man is to hear, "Well, I told you what I wanted" or "You should know by now. We have been together forever." Let me tell you right now, don't play that stupid stuff. Men just get more annoyed when women expect us to know what is going on in their minds.

When you play that game, you just get men angry and they will walk away. This doesn't solve anything and just ruins the situation. When it comes to your relationships, don't play this game and just tell men what you want or why this is the case. It will lead to a lot less arguments and annoyances. Women say they want a man to communicate in the relationship. Well ladies, men want the same from you. So, open your mouth, let the words fly, and make sure everything is clear. It will lead to a lot less headaches down the road.

CHAPTER SIX
Dating When You Are Shy And Or Socially Awkward

Talking to new people is totally awkward for most people. When you add in the emotional aspect and the possibilities of dating and long-term relationships into the mix, the thought of walking up to or even being approached by someone interested in you can be totally debilitating.

When I was in school, I never went up to anyone and told them I liked them. Even when I heard whispers in the halls that so and so had a crush on me, I would just shrivel up in my own shell and enter my own world. I think that this is one reason I became a writer. When I could enter my own world and have total control of the events that I created, it made life easier.

When I grew up, however, I had to deal with several deaths. I had to deal with the death of my father, I had to deal with the death of a friend's child, and I had to deal with the death of one of a significant other. All of these happened within the span of a year. So, in my mind, I was on the fence if I were to ever find love again. Then, I found myself in a life and death situation where I could have died. Thankfully, I survived but it left me in a mental state where I could have gone either direction. After a long time of feeling bad about myself and my situation, I suddenly hit rock bottom and decided, "Forget it." I am not going to let the actions or inactions of other determine my fate. So, after that I took control back of my life, I am now in long-term relationship going on six years, have two children, and we will be married by the time this book is published.

The reason that I told you this story about me is to let you know that there is no fear in life. Fear is a state of mind left over from early evolution. When facing fear, we have two ways of dealing with it. Either let it control you or you control it. When dating and meeting others, I personally feel that you need to have a life changing event that switches on that switch in your brain and tells you there is no fear. You need to say, "Forget it" and take a chance. The worst thing that can happen is you will be right where you are now. The best thing that can happen is you find true love and happiness.

Making the First Move

So, if you are socially awkward or unsure of your situation, how would you make the first move? Well, there are several ways to do this. First, you don't want to build up the situation in your head. This is where most people get all caught up and will freeze themselves with fear. Don't let your minds freeze you up like men let their male parts say stupid things.

When making your first move, you want to be subtle. You want to slip into a situation where it looks like you are not slipping into a situation. For example, if you are at a bar or another social event and you see someone look to see if there is a chair next to them that you can sit in, ask if anyone is sitting there and if they aren't, sit down.

The next thing is to show that you aren't interested. You want to sit down, order a drink, and then take out your phone and look at it. You want to look at Facebook, play *Candy Crush*, or whatever. Then you want to pick up on something subtle he is doing and make a comment. This will be your ice breaker into the conversation. From there, just talk to them like normal. If you have a spark, move the conversation to a private table. If not, have your phone set to ring, answer it, make an excuse, and leave.

Travel in Packs

Women are famous for this. When going out in social situations, take a woman or two. Men do it, they just call them wing men. When you take a woman, she can be your wing woman or whatever you want to call her. When you have someone with you, it is easier to get into and out of situations. For example, if you are afraid to talk to someone, your friend can go up and initiate the conversation. If you want to get out of the situation, your friend can jump in and say that she wants to go home or there is something that needs to be taken care of.

When you travel in packs, you have extra security as well as someone watching your back. In the dating world, men are crazy. Women are just as crazy, but you will typically find out if a man is crazy earlier on in the relationship. Women typically will go nuts a few days or weeks later. Sorry women, but it is true.

Just Chill

At the end of the day, you just want to chill. When starting to date, just go with the flow, don't go into anything with preconceived thoughts or actions and don't go to places you normally wouldn't go to. For example, if you are not a drinker and don't want to meet a man in that environment then don't go there. If you want someone who has your values and what you like to do then go to a place of interest and see what you can find. You never know, you might meet a friend of a friend you may never have met.

It will Happen When It Happens

Don't go crazy and get depressed if you don't find Mr. Right ten minutes into your search. It took me over thirty years before I found the person I was supposed to be with. The relationship I was in before I met my spouse to be is almost the same as my previous relationship. The person I was with prior had a lot of the same traits I found attractive, but the underlying emotional connection are different.

So, just go with it and let it happen. I firmly believe that all our life paths are already in motion. Sooner or later, you will meet that person. Just let it happen and grab on with both hands when it does.

Don't go in Search for Love

Now, I know this probably sounds like I am contradicting myself but here me out. When people join dating sites, match making networks, or join single cruise clubs, they are focused on finding love. This is a mistake.

When it comes to finding love, there is nothing to find. Love is not a physical thing that you can just go up on eBay or Shopify and add to a shopping cart. Love is something that needs to start with a spark, then from that spark, a small flame needs to grow and from that flame, a roaring fire. Love is something that can't even be explained. Why do you love someone has been a question asked by scientists since the beginning of time.

If you were to put love and the emotions that it represents into a physical object, what would it be? If love were a physical object then it can easily be replaced, altered, and understood. However, this is not the case.

Another question you will have to ask yourself is if love were tangible, why is it so hard to find? Also, if two people had love standing right in front of them wouldn't that love be equal? One person couldn't have more love for another person. And no one could also fall out of love.

Therefore, you don't want to have the preconceptions in your mind that you are going to find love. The secret is to love is to allow it to find you. If you were to ask couples that have been together for twenty, thirty years how they fell in love, most of them will tell you that it just happened one day.

Therefore, you don't want to go in search of it. Just let the universe know that you are ready for love and it will find you. Trust me, it works. This is how it happened to me.

CHAPTER SEVEN
Sizing Up Your Possible Mate

Alright, we have gotten through all the hard stuff. We have figured out who we are and what we want out of a relationship with another person, we have a good understanding of what a man wants and how he wants to be treated; we have talked about social situations and how to deal with them. Now for the big moment. What to do to ensure that the man you are going to give the time of day to and possibly make a lifelong commitment to is worth your time and energy.

The First Impression

When it comes to dating, they say you can never make a second first impression. This is true in many aspects of dating and in life in general. When we come together for the first time, the universe has done so for a reason. Since the beginning of time, atoms, molecules, and cosmic dust have been lowing aimlessly through space. The events of the past have been working towards this specific moment in time. The actions of your parents, grandparents, great grandparents, outcomes in war, and even what you ordered for dinner last night have played a role in this exact moment of you and this person coming together in this specific moment in time. So, what are you going to do with it?

Wow, that was a little dramatic, wasn't it? Well, it was meant to be. For you, see if you think about first impressions and how the universe really puts things together. You will probably go nuts.

Seriously though. When it comes to first impressions, you really need to make sure that they are memorable. This doesn't mean that you walk around with a full orchestral band or jump around in a Spiderman outfit. What it means is that you really need to just be you in these situations. If you are not you then what is the point.

When thinking about first impressions with women, men need to make sure they don't act like a jerk. Women have great selective memory when it comes to these things. Women will remember the shirt men were wearing, the cologne they had on, and even the music that was playing in the background. The reason for this is that women want to remember the love of their lives and without knowing if you are it, they will remember it just in case.

Attitude Towards Life

Women don't want downers. They want a man that is positive and has a plan. When women are looking for men they want to know it will be a long lasting positive experience. If you are someone who has a good job or is working towards a good job, likes what they are doing, isn't down about something that happened at work or in life, then women will pick up on this and become more accretive of men and their actions. If they are negative, don't care and just want to be left alone then this will be picked up as well and it won't typically turn out to be a good experience.

Friends and Family

Women want to know how you are with friends and family. One of the biggest questions women will want to know is how he treats his mother. If a man treats his mother with love and respect then it is a good indicator that she will be treated with love and respect.

How do they interact with their friends? Does he have any friends? How do they act? When looking at a man's friends, you can tell a lot about their actions. If you see that they hang out with a lot of people that are calm and professional, then you can assume that he is calm and professional. If you see that he hangs out with a lot of questionable people, then you can assume that he is into a lot of questionable activities or at least will be exposed to these activities at some point.

Anger

How does he deal with stress and anger? Is he someone who is quick to anger and react or is he more laid back and mellow? Is he a push over when it comes to be bullied or will he stand up and take care of the situation when it presents itself? This is a very big deal and can be a red flag in the relationship.

If a man gets angry and is quick to lash out physically, then it can be a sign that he could lash out and become physical or violent towards you. Is he someone who lets people push him around? This is not a good thing either. If you find yourself in a situation that you need to be stood up for or protected, will he do it. Now, this doesn't mean going out there and physically fighting everyone that threatens you. This can be as simple as standing up to someone in defense of your woman.

For example, if you are out and someone makes a rude comment or says something that you know is wrong, will you stand up for her and take her side or you will step back and take the side of others even though you know she is right?

When it comes to anger and dealing with situations like these, a woman really needs to know that you will stand up and be a man. She doesn't want a bully or a possessive jackass, but she does want to know that you are on her side and that this is an "our" relationship type of situation.

Kids

Where are you with kids? Do you like kids? Do you want kids? Does she have kids?

Women and kids are a very touchy and sensitive subject. When first starting out in the relationship, a woman will be looking to see how you handle yourself around other kids. They will see if you like kids, if you are friendly, talk to them on their level, are quick to anger, and a slew of other points. If the woman is looking to have kids or start a family, they are looking first and foremost if you are someone that would be a good fit for that situation. If not, you don't have a prayer in starting a relationship.

Money and Finances

They say money is the root of all evil. In the United States alone, more and more families and couples are torn apart over money and finances. This can be brought on by many factors:

1. He doesn't make enough money

2. He spends more money than he needs to and on things he doesn't need

3. He snaps at a woman if she spends money without asking

4. He wants to be in control of the money more and she wants more freedom

These are just a few points when it comes to money. I am sure you can add to this list without even having to half try, but for the most part, these are the top four. When getting into a serious relationship or considering if this is Mr. Right then you need to have the money talk. You want to set rules and terms on who pays for what, if the money is equal, if he is going to work, and if she is going to stay home and much more.

In life situations, change and the amount of money that is brought in compared to what goes out will forever be in flux. Therefore, budgets need to be created and kept to. If you can't make a budget, talk about how the budget is to be spent and agree to how much you will put away for a rainy day. If you don't, the relationship will be strained, and money and finances will be the reason.

Future Goals

Goals are vital in life. What are your goals in education? What are your goals in a home, car, employment, retirement, kids? When determining if this is going to me Mr. Right, these questions need to be asked, answered, and reevaluated on a regular basis. When you enter a relationship, the relationship will change. When you reach a goal, new goals will take its place. Therefore, you want to have time set aside each month, three months, and year to talk about these. Remember, communication is key. If you can't talk about it, you need to figure out why.

Mr. Right Now

When starting out and determining if this is going to be Mr. Right, don't stress yourself. In the beginning, he doesn't have to be Mr. Right. You can defiantly be in search of Mr. Right Now, and just have some fun. However, if Mr. Right Now changes, you need to be prepared.

Engaging in Likeminded Activities

When dating, you will want to figure out fun and interesting things to do. One way to test if the person you are with will be a good life partner is to put them to the test and have them engage with you in your favorite activity. For example, if you like running then you will want to see how you enjoy running together. If you like climbing mountains, white water rafting, camping or whatever, you will want to do these activities with them. When you engage in these activities, you will start to form bonds. You will also see if you and the other person can work together on these activities as well as how they will react to losing as well as winning.

When you engage in sports or healthy competition, will the other person let you win or take control and beat you? If they win, will they rub your nose in it or be a graceful winner? If they lose, will they go stomping off like a little baby? It is when you start challenging and engaging your relationship with factors that will be part of your life long adventure will you determine and understand if this is the Mr. Right or Mr. Right Now. Have fun and throw in a few curb balls as well. It will be fun to see if you are really meant for each other.

Engaging in SEX!

The final thing I wanted to bring up would be the first time you and your partner engage in sex. If you are going to be in this relationship for the long haul, you want to make sure that he isn't a bad lay. One of the worst things in any relationship is finding out that your partner isn't good at sex, wants to do things that you don't want to do, or is uncomfortable doing as well as their sexual appetite. In many relationships, finding out about your sexual compatibility will be the deciding factor if you are going to move this to the next level and be life partners. So, when you decide to have sex for the first time, you don't want to be shy or timid. You don't want to do things that you are uncomfortable with and you don't want to put yourself into a situation that will make him or her expect that the act you just performed will be an all the time thing.

So, when engaging in sex for the first time, plan it out, make it hot and dirty, and don't hesitate to be you. This will be your first sexual experience with him, so make it the best that it can be for you. If you are not compatible, it may be your last.

Rinse and Repeat

Finally, don't hesitate to date multiple people. Dating isn't an instant win at the casino. It will take going through a few lemons to find that perfect someone. Don't be afraid to kick a few around and see what falls out.

CHAPTER EIGHT
Dating Advice for New and
Unexperienced Daters

In this chapter, I am going to give you some dating advice and even touch on some areas we mentioned already in the book. When starting to date, had a lot of bad dates, or just feel you are unexperienced, these tips will help you out.

Tip #1 – Respect Yourself Over Everything Else

If you don't respect yourself and show it then no one else will either. Men want a confident woman that knows what she wants and isn't afraid to go for it. This means that you don't want to flaunt your sexuality, act trashy, talk dirty, or swear like a man. You want to dress nice, be yourself, and hold your head up high. If you have poor hygiene, look down at your feet, and present yourself in a way that isn't you then you are staring off on the wrong foot. Respect yourself, be your own person and that will be the most attractive thing you can ever do.

Tip #2 – Keep Life Simple

When dating men, they don't want to know your life story, what baggage you are carrying with you from your past, and how much work you can possibly be. When dating, you want to go into the situation with a clean slate. Don't go into it with preconceived notions of falling in love, having a thousand kids, living in a mansion, and sitting on your butt like Peggy Bundy. Keep the first impression simple, learn about each other, and just see what happens.

Tip #3 – Don't Dominate the Conversation

When meeting someone, don't dominate the conversation. Many men are out to impress you, so they will want to talk. Let them talk and when asked a question, give responses, ask your own questions, and tell stories. This is supposed to be a fun getting to know you time in your life. Take advantage of it and keep the conversation even.

Tip #4 – It's Not About Sex

When starting to date, don't jump into sex or talking sexy. Now, if it moves in that direction and you are both up for it, I can't tell you no. However, if this is going to be a Mr. Right not a Mr. Right Now situation, then take it slow. Don't talk dirty or tell dirty jokes. Don't talk about past boyfriends and don't let him talk about past girlfriends. These conversations can be put off till a later date. If this is going to be Mr. Right, then there will be plenty of time for sex.

Tip #5 – Keep Alcohol and Drugs out of the Date

When going on a date, it is common to go to a restaurant and have a few cocktails with dinner. This is okay on the third of fourth date, but on the first date, you want to really consider keeping alcohol and other drugs out of the situation. This can lead to bad judgment and situations you don't want to find yourself in. If you do go to dinner, try to get something you can handle or limit yourself to one drink. Another thing is that you don't want to leave your drink unattended. There are a lot of crazy people out there and you don't want to take the chance of the unthinkable happening.

Tip #6 – Be Spontaneous

Men like it when you take control and know what you want. If you sit there and let them make all the decisions or act like you don't care, then men will think you are not into the date and will send the wrong signal. When you have broken the ice, it is a good idea to speak up and share what is on your mind. Ask them to dance in the restaurant, have him come in close for a selfie, or go somewhere that you never would have gone like miniature golf. When you take the initiative and do something spontaneous even if you planned it ahead of time, the guy will take it as a sign that you are cool and are interested in a possible relationship. So, be spontaneous and unexpected. It will pay off in the long run.

Tip #7 - Don't Introduce Them to your Family Too Quickly

When it comes to dating, you don't want to move too quickly and introduce them to your parents. Now, this can also be a touchy subject. When is the best time to introduce him to mom and dad? The same goes for him as well. When do you really want to meet his mom, dad, forty-six brothers and sisters, and cat fluffy? Do you really want to go to his childhood home and see his bedroom where God knows what went on in there?

You will want to introduce each other to your respective families after a month or two has gone by and you feel that you really want to take the relationship into a relationship. When you are ready to meet the family, it will feel right. Until then, just have your secret guy all to yourself.

Tip #8 – Have an Escape Plan

When starting out, you want to have an escape plan. This is for safety and to get out of a bad date. One thing that you can do is have a friend follow you to the location and hide in the shadows. They can be at another table in a restaurant or bar, a stranger in the movie theater, or just someone on phone standby. When dating, you never know what you are going to get yourself into so make sure that you have a clear exit strategy and even check in a few times with a bathroom break.

Tip #9 – Start your Dates Early

There is no rule that you must have a night date. You can setup your date to be on a weekend or even a lunch date. When you set up your dates to be earlier in the day, you not only have more options of things to do, but you can easily have an excuse to cut the date short or use the phrase, "Well it's getting late. I need to go home and get ready for work tomorrow."

Tip #10 – Never Settle

You don't want to settle for the first person you come across. There are many fish in the sea as it were. Take your time, see what feels right, and don't be afraid to switch it up once and awhile. If it was meant to be, it will be. The universe will put you together with the perfect person for you. Just be open and willing to accept them.

Tip #11 – Make your Personal Boundaries Known

When you start dating and opening yourself up to others, it is important that you know where your personal boundaries are. One of the things that happen when you start dating is your emotions and sexual desires will start to play hard with your inhibitions and decisions. When you start dating someone, you will want to let them and know when it would be good for you to get kissed, hold hands, hug and engage in other forms of physical activity. When you start dating a man, they will generally move a little faster than you will and as such put you into situations that you may not feel comfortable being in or add alcohol that will lessen your inhibitions.

If you make your personal boundaries known and where you stand on specific areas of your own personal body, then there will be no question about inappropriate behavior. Starting new relationships and meeting new people, engaging in new experiences is something that everyone should do. Just set your boundaries and rules upfront and things will move smoother.

Tip #12 – Use Tools to Build Powerful Relationships

Like everything else in life, you will want to build up a tool base. Depending on you and your own personal habits your tools may look different. One tool that you will want to have is a small book of emergency numbers. These can be taxi numbers or numbers to friends and family. When you have these numbers, you can keep them hidden on you in case you lose your phone, or the battery goes dead. This way, if you find yourself in a situation without your phone, you have numbers that you can call or have others call for you.

Another tool would be some hidden money. When going out on a date, you will always want to have enough money for a taxi, phone call, and an emergency. What you will want to do each month is take a few dollars out of your paycheck and slide them into a hidden place in your phone case or small coin purse. When you have a hidden twenty always, you know that you can make your way home or at least arrange with someone to get you to where you will be safe. The last thing you want to do is find yourself in a situation where you have no cash and having to get home without a ride.

Tip #13 – Take Control of your Life

When dating, the first thing you want to do is be in a good place in your own life. This is very important. If you are not in control of your own life, then bringing someone else into your life will not end well. If you don't have a job, car, money, or an education to help you get these things, then bringing someone else into your life will not end well either. If you are personally stable, you will help balance the relationship.

Don't let others control you. This is another vital part to having a great dating relationship. When you get into a relationship, you may feel pressured to do what the other person wants to do all the time. This is not a good sign of a healthy relationship. You want to be in control of your part. You want to suggest places to go, people to hang out with, and even take charge of paying for the bill. We are in a new age of dating, women, you can pay the bill as well. I know that is taboo, but equal rights mean equal responsibilities.

When dating, you will want to reflect on these tips. As you get more experience in dating and finding what you want as well as what you don't want, you will be able to add more tips and tricks to your dating toolbox.

CHAPTER NINE
Meghan's Story

Meghan grew up in a small town in Florida. She was a happy child living with her two brothers and cat Junior. Her parents didn't really have a lot of money with her dad working as a delivery driver and her mother being a stay at home mom. Even though things were tight at times, Meghan and her two brothers never wanted for anything.

As Meghan got older, she began to develop into an attractive young lady. She was about five feet eight, long blonde hair, and radiant blue eyes. A typical all-American Florida girl. One day when she was coming home from school, she was astonished to see her mother sitting on the back porch by the pool crying with a drink in her hand. Tossing her book bag to the side, she ran to her mother's side, placed a hand on her knee, and asked what was going on.

Taking a sip of her vodka and water, her mother stared blankly out at the pool before uttering the one thing that I believed would never happen. You see, it was made known that my father, the man I looked up to, admired and wanted to be like when I grew up, was having an affair with another woman. My mother told me that the affair had been going on for over five years right under our noses. It seems that when my father would go off on these long trips, he was going to this woman's house.

Gripping onto my mother's hand even tighter, I began to cry myself. As I held my mother, I began to wonder what it was like to be really in love. If my parents, people I have believed were in love all my life could have this happen to them, then what hope could I possibly have?

Several Years Later....

I was now twenty-one years old and out on my own. I have moved to Daytona Beach Florida now and have found myself a small house on the beach to rent. I have a job working at the local hotel and was making good money. The tourist season was in high swing, so I was busier than ever taking care of guests and seeing to my other duties.

One day while I was finishing up a phone call, a tall, dark, and handsome man came up to the desk where I was working. I had just finished up a phone call and didn't recognize him for a moment or two. When I did notice him, I raised my head and let out one of my typical smiles. "Yes sir, how can I help you?"

The man was tall, about five-nine or six feet. He had dark flowing black hair, and a little bit of a five o'clock shadow which I have always found sexy in a man. He was wearing a white dress shirt, blue shorts, and sneakers. When my eyes met his, I was suddenly and unexpectedly interested.

"Yes, I hate to bother you, but I have been sitting over there admiring you for a while now. I don't want to appear to be forward, but I was wondering if you would be interested in having a drink with me after you get off work."

Forcing myself not to take a step back in case he might take my intentions wrong, I fought with myself not to bite my lower lip.

"Umm..." I struggled to find the words." Before I was able to answer, he jumped in saving me from myself.

"I know I may seem a little forward and I am sure there are probably some policies in place from employees dating guests, but…"

As he continued his pickup line, I found myself flustered and blurting out "NO." Shocked at what I had said, the man lowered his head in shocking disappointment. "No, I don't mean no to the drink," I corrected trying to redeem myself, "I meant no to there being rules about staff dating guests, I mean having a drink." I need to keep watching myself.

Turning his attention back towards me with renewed optimism, he smiled this amazing smile and said, "So, is that a yes on the drink?"

I hesitated for only a moment just to make him wait in anticipation for my reply. Then when I felt he waited long enough, I let out a giant grin and a confirming YES.

"Great, what time do you get off work?" he asked leaning in closer to my desk.

"Seven thirty," I replied.

"Great," tapping his finger on the desk, he shot me back a gorgeous smile, "I will pick you up here then." And with that, he walked away out of the lobby.

Standing there speechless over what had just happened, I had totally forgotten that Sarah was standing at the other counter listening to every word that had transpired. Still in my trance, I was suddenly returned to reality with the words, "OOH girl, you had better tap you some of that before I do."

Darting my attention in her direction, my jaw was almost hitting the floor. I had to quickly recompose myself when another guest began to walk up to my desk.

I had spent the rest of the day dealing with guests as best I could. Every time someone new came to my desk, I couldn't help but relive the encounter with that sexy guest. As I was finishing setting up an early morning wakeup call, the dark-haired stranger approached my station once again. This time he was wearing light brown slacks and a navy-blue shirt.

"Are you ready?" he asked as he came up to my desk and leaned up against it, palms down on the glass with drumming fingers. It took me a minute to regain my composure before I was able to answer him.

"Oh, yes, just give me a minute to punch out." With a bright smile I gave him one more eye candy stare before taking a step back turning to the right and walking down the hall. When I reached the employee break room, I found myself standing up against the wall pulling my shirt in and out to create some wind. Letting out a deep breath, I composed myself, punched my time card and when I was ready, went back out into the lobby and headed to the hotel bar with my date.

The lighting in the hotel bar were dim and somewhat romantic. As I walked over the threshold, my date gestures to the bar.

Walking to an empty seat, I get comfortable at a stool where he sits beside me. "Evening Meghan, what can I get for you?" John the bartender asks.

"My usual, vodka and water," turning his attention to the man, "And for you, sir?"

"Rum and coke." With a nod, John walks back and forth behind the bar as the man positions his stool so that it was closer to me.

"You know, I don't even know your name?" Meghan chuckled with a little girlish laugh.

"It's Brian," the man replied getting comfortable next to her.

Letting out a little chuckle, Meghan brushes her hair back a little and gives Brian a smile. A moment later, John returns with her drink, places it in front of her, and finishes adding the coke to Brian's drink a moment later. With both drinks in hand, the newly formed couple raise their glasses and Brian makes a toast.

"To a great evening," Meghan replies with a nod as the two clink glasses, lock eyes, and take a sip.

"So, what do you do Brian?" Meghan asks with intent interest.

"I am a computer technician. I go around the country fixing computers in banks, hotels, and restaurants. I love to travel and meet new people. I am here in Florida for another day then I have to fly out to California."

"Wow, interesting. I have always wanted to travel, but never got around to it. My father left us when we were younger, and we had to pretty much fend for ourselves. My mother had gone into a deep depression after our father left and began to drink heavily. After a few months, we were forced to sell our house and get our own apartments since she drank herself to death. "

Sitting there listening intently, Brian raised an eyebrow, took a sip of his drink, and then returned the glass to the table. "Really, that must have been rough on you," he replied.

"Yes, a little, but everything seems to have worked out alright. I have a great job here at the hotel. It doesn't pay a lot, but I get to meet interesting people." Taking another sip of her drink, Meghan places the glass back down on the bar, rubbed her hands up and down on her black skirt, and took a quick glance around the bar.

Brian looks at Meghan and asks, "Are you looking for someone?" Darting her attention back to Brian, Meghan runs her finger through her hair, tucking a small clump behind her ear and laughs.

"Oh, no, I just like to check out the bar to see the different people that come in here. I have always been a people watcher ever since I was a kid. I guess that is why I took a job in a hotel. With all the different people that come in and out of here, you can't but wonder what their stories are."

Looking around the bar again, Meghan points out a family sitting at booth number five. "You see that couple over there with the small kids. I bet they are going to be going to Disneyworld. The young boy is wearing Mickey ears and the girl a princess dress. "

Brian looks over at the table and smiles. "It is great to see kids having a good time. It brings me hope that I will be a great father one day. Do you want kids?"

Meghan turns her attention back towards Brian and shrugs her shoulders. "I don't know. I haven't thought about it really. Ever since my dad left, I really haven't thought much about what I really wanted in a family. This is the first date I had in over three years. I just haven't put too much thought or effort into myself and my future. Just going through the motions, I guess."

Taking another sip of drink Brian takes a quick glance at his watch. "Oh dear, have we been here talking this long. I must be ready to catch an early plane in the morning. Motioning to John, Brian hands the man his credit card and asks him to close out his tab. Turning back to Meghan he replies, "Well Meghan, I hate to run off like this, but I do have a lot of stuff to do before the morning. It was a pleasure talking to you and I hope that when I get back this way we can do dinner or something."

Giving Brian a smile, she shakes his hand. "I would like that." Signing the credit card receipt, Brian puts his copy into his wallet, downs the last remaining remanence of his drink, gives Meghan a hug, and walks out the door. A moment later, Meghan turns towards John and gives him a slight huff.

"Is everything okay?"

"I don't know. I guess I am not really good at dating." She says twirling the ice in her drink.

"Why do you say that?" asked John.

"We were only here for ten minutes and he had to go to bed. Said he had an early flight in the morning." Taking a quick glance at his watch it reads 8:00. Without saying another word, John goes behind the bar, mixes up another drink, and hands it to Meghan.

"On the house."

Breaking down the date

Now that you have read our story and gone on this date with Meghan and Brian, I want you to go through the entire date from start to finish. I want you to put yourself in Meghan's position as well as in Brian's position. When you do, I want you to take notes in your notebook as to what each one did right and what each one did wrong. From there, I want you to write down what you would have done differently in this situation. This is a learning experience and is based on a typical first date situation.

Ask yourself the following questions.

What happened before the date and what could Meghan done differently to better prepare herself. She had stated that she hasn't dated in a while, so what do you think of her bringing along a wing man or wing woman as it were on the date? If she didn't want to bring one along, maybe she could have had her friend sitting in the bar watching the date or maybe come in for a drink after her shift.

When the date started, what did Brian do right and what did he do wrong?

When talking about herself, should Meghan have brought up all the details of her past?

When Brian asked her about children and told her that he wanted to be a father, do you think he should have brought up that information so early in the meeting or should he have waited?

When Meghan was looking around the room, should she have been doing that or should she have been putting her full attention towards Brian?

When Meghan brought up the fact that her mother began drinking after her father left and Meghan was drinking the same drink, do you think a red flag was set off in Brian's head that Meghan could have baggage that he isn't ready or willing to deal with either now or in the future?

At what point of the date do you believe Brian was "Hell no, I got to go" in his mind? Where would you have called it quits or would you still be there sticking it out to see if you could just get a little sex before you left and never returned?

The world is a strange place. We meet people at random and find ourselves in situations that we never expected. It is amazing that men and women get together at all and form relationships. Wouldn't it just be easier to have sex and move on?

I hope you took something away from this story and will use the idea to build your own date. Go ahead and see what you would have done.

CONCLUSION

When it comes to dating, there is no right or wrong answers. Life is filled with different people, different beliefs, and different ways of doing things. In the rule book on dating, there are no rules. It is all a matter of trial and error, taking chances, and allowing yourself to be open and accepting of what the universe is sending your way.

In this book, I have attempted to give you a guide that you can follow and adapt to your own specific needs. I want you to understand that these rules, tips, tricks, and nuggets of advice are written in stone. Many of these have been taken from my own personal experiences when it came to dating. I want you to learn from my mistakes and my successes and with every chance encounter, blind date, and secret admirer, you find yourself and your Prince Charming.

Thank you for taking this journey with me and I hope that your next dating adventure will be the best one yet!